IF I REALLY WANTED TO
LOSE WEIGHT,
I WOULD . . .

Honor Books

Tulsa, Oklahoma

If I Really Wanted to Lose Weight, I Would . . .
ISBN 1-56292-566-0
Copyright © 2000 by Honor Books
P. O. Box 55388
Tulsa, Oklahoma 74155

Manuscript prepared by W. B. Freeman Concepts, Inc.
Tulsa, Oklahoma.

Introduction

You've moved from the seriously deficient grapefruit, hard-boiled egg, and liquid food diets to the measure-anything-you-set-on-a-plate plan. Yet, despite your best efforts, you find yourself hungry, irritable, obsessed with food, and wondering, *Is this worth it?*

So many people are looking for the right solution only to find frustration and fleeting improvement. It seems the only options are to try yet another, perhaps more drastic, diet, or give up all together. And you should give up. You should give up any temporary, crazy diet that promises success in a short time but doesn't prepare you for the long-haul (namely, the rest of your life).

A more balanced approach includes easy-to-manage baby steps that lead to change in thought, focus, and habits. A new lifestyle is adopted, in some ways without even realizing it, bringing with it weight loss and so much more. Remember, the most important aspect of any plan is the ability to keep the weight off over time.

In this book, we've provided tips, insights, and inspiration to help you make those important lifestyle changes. Leave diets in the dust and don't look back. Walk bravely toward a plan that will make you a success story for life.

Lose Weight,

I Would . . .

Ask for
God's help.

*I can do everything through
him who gives me strength.*
—Philippians 4:13

Even those people who feel comfortable about bringing their difficulties to God often seem reluctant to ask for His help when it comes to diet and food issues. That's a shame because anyone who has struggled with them knows just how tough they can be. "I just don't have any willpower," is an often-heard dieter's lament.

Everyone feels weak at times—if not with food, then with any number of other tough temptations. The Bible tells us that God will not allow us to be tempted beyond what we can endure and He will always provide a way out. God not only can, but will help you win the weight-loss challenge.

Strength is ours for the asking.

Lose Weight,

I Would . . .

Get key
starting
numbers.

௸

*Be sure you put your feet in the
right place. Then stand firm.*
—Abraham Lincoln

Before you commit yourself to stand firm until the weight comes off, pause to collect all the pertinent numbers related to your health—blood pressure, cholesterol count (both HDL and LDL), blood chemistry breakdown, and weight. Such a checkup will also serve to isolate any specific problems you may need to address with a physician.

This will help you establish a clear benchmark in your mind and alert you to any potential complications brought about by increased exercise and a change in diet. Check again in six months to see if you are making progress. Be faithful, and you should see numbers that truly make you feel good!

Know where you stand before you start.

Lose Weight,

I Would . . .

Ask my doctor to help me set realistic goals.

❧

The beginning is the most important part of the work.
—Plato

One excellent means of establishing realistic, safe goals is to check with your doctor. Ask him or her to help you establish the right goal weight, taking into consideration your bone structure, age, family history, and any special medical needs you may have.

This information is critical to the success of your weight-loss plan because it will help you determine how quickly you should lose pounds and what your ideal weight should be. It's a big mistake to base your goal on media images of body size. The perfect weight is different with every person.

No army goes into battle without a medical corps.

Lose Weight,

I Would . . .

Make every bite count.

*Now this is what the LORD
Almighty says:
"Give careful thought
to your ways."*
—Haggai 1:5

Have you ever found yourself grazing at the hors d'oeuvres table, catching up on the latest with friends, hardly aware of what and how much you are eating? Are potato chips trusted companions in times of boredom or stress?

For so many, habitual, almost unconscious, eating can add thousands of extra calories, and many unwanted pounds, but never really satisfy your hunger. Identify the situations and foods that trigger this type of eating, and take steps to change the way you respond to them. Choose instead to be aware of how you are eating, and make every bite count—find food you truly enjoy and do just that—*enjoy* a small portion consciously.

Weight modification requires behavior modification.

Lose Weight,

I Would . . .

Stop eating the
moment I feel full.

*Prudence means practical
common sense, taking the
trouble to think out what you
are doing and what is
likely to become of it.*
—C. S. Lewis

Our brains have been designed to receive a message from the stomach when we've reached capacity. It's a "whoa, that's enough" signal, which many of us, through years of practice, have learned to ignore.

We have retrained our brain to obey the familiar admonition, "Finish everything on your plate." We put too much on our plates, and then we feel compelled to eat it all. Don't be afraid to leave a few bites, and practice listening for that little voice in your head. It may be muffled, but it's still there. It will tell you when it's time to put the fork down.

Listen to your brain—it tells the truth about how much food you REALLY need.

Lose Weight,

I Would . . .

Learn more about how the body uses food.

I do not feel that the same God who has endowed us with sense, reason, and intellect has intended us to forego their use.
—Galileo Galilei

Do you know which foods are fattening and why? What is required for overall good nutrition? What constitutes a balanced diet? What do various nutrients do for the body? Which foods are rich in which nutrients? What foods trigger your metabolism? What combinations of food accelerate weight loss?

A responsible weight-loss plan should always include education about healthful eating. Don't rely on books that present fad approaches to foods or offer a "miracle" food supplement. Choose information sources that emphasize nutrients, a combination of exercise and eating, and a balanced menu. Just like in any other aspect of life, knowledge is an important tool for success.

Information can be your best weight-loss aid—learn it and use it!

Lose Weight,

I Would . . .

Have a weight-loss buddy.

ক্ষ্ব

Two are better than one, because
they have a good return for
their work: If one falls down,
his friend can help him up.
—Ecclesiastes 4:9,10

Nationally known weight-loss organizations get results. That's because they've discovered that personal support is a key ingredient in successful weight-loss programs. Having regular checkpoints for accountability to a friend or group can make the critical difference. Some people *can* do it alone, but most find that it's extremely helpful to know someone special is watching with interest as you weigh in.

So find a friend and ask him or her to seriously consider making a commitment to you as you embark on your weight-loss plan. Then when you feel tempted to throw in the towel, call your buddy. A calm voice of reason is usually all you really need to stay the course.

Good friends always want the best for us.

Lose Weight,

I Would . . .

Exercise more.

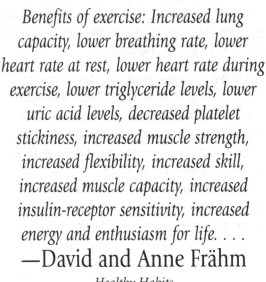

*Benefits of exercise: Increased lung
capacity, lower breathing rate, lower
heart rate at rest, lower heart rate during
exercise, lower triglyceride levels, lower
uric acid levels, decreased platelet
stickiness, increased muscle strength,
increased flexibility, increased skill,
increased muscle capacity, increased
insulin-receptor sensitivity, increased
energy and enthusiasm for life. . . .*

—David and Anne Frähm

Healthy Habits

Despite its benefits, we can all think of a hundred reasons why we can't exercise in a given day—time, fatigue, inconvenience. Nevertheless, weight loss actually has a simple formula: LESS INPUT OF CALORIES + GREATER OUTPUT OF ENERGY = WEIGHT LOSS.

Trying to lose weight without exercising is like trying to climb a mountain without training. Brief workouts—walking, jogging, swimming, or lifting weights—should be added to your daily routine. Find activities you enjoy and start slowly. Your body will quickly begin to convert fat to muscle. Over time, your metabolism will actually change, which means that keeping the weight off will be easier.

Twenty minutes of exercise a day can mean the difference between "fab" and flab.

Post incremental goals on the refrigerator door.

*Let your eyes look straight
ahead, fix your gaze
directly before you.*
—Proverbs 4:25

You didn't gain your excess weight in a day, and you won't lose all the weight you desire to lose in a week or month—perhaps even a year. Give yourself some short-term goals you can focus on and reach quickly. You'll feel an ongoing sense of satisfaction, and you will be more motivated to stay on your weight-loss plan.

Set your short-term goals with caution. Two pounds a week is generally a safe and realistic pace for weight-loss. And just think, two pounds a week for a year is more than a hundred pounds! Staying focused on the short-term goals will keep you from becoming overwhelmed.

⟨❧⟩

Small steps can add up to big strides.

Lose Weight,

I Would . . .

Take the stairs.

❧

Physical fitness means energetically performing daily tasks to the best of your ability without getting exhausted. [It] also means that you still have energy to do the fun stuff that you love so much.

—Bodies In Motion . . . Minds at Rest fitness web site

The more you move, the more you lose! So it makes sense to cut out some of the labor-saving conveniences in your life and opt for exerting renewable human energy. Use a rake instead of a leaf blower, a push mower instead of a power mower. Walk instead of riding a cart around the golf course. Choose the parking place farthest away from the store. Do exercises while talking on the telephone. Walk rather than drive to nearby destinations and pick up your pace.

A little more effort and a few more minutes taken for activity in your daily routine can yield significant benefits. Move it and lose it.

Add a little effort into your everyday events. It's exercise in disguise!

Lose Weight,

I Would . . .

Reward myself for meeting goals.

ॐ

The reward of a thing well done is to have done it.
—Ralph Waldo Emerson

When you meet an incremental goal in your weight-loss plan, you can feel good simply knowing you've accomplished your objective. However, going one step further and doing something tangible for yourself marks a milestone and gives you the added motivation to continue on with your plan.

Buy a dress in your new reduced size, take a day trip or a get-away with your favorite person, buy tickets to a special event or game, or buy yourself a huge bouquet of your favorite flowers—just try to stay away from the double-chocolate cheesecake reward. The more you reward yourself with nonfood rewards, the more likely you will be to avoid rewarding yourself with food in the future.

Reward yourself with life's sweetness, but not with sweets.

Lose Weight,

I Would . . .

Refuse to give up if I slip and binge.

✥

Brothers, I do not consider myself yet to have taken hold of it. But one thing I do: Forgetting what is behind and straining toward what is ahead, I press on toward the goal to win the prize for which God has called me heavenward in Christ Jesus.

—Philippians 3:13,14

Managing your weight takes practice to make perfect. Every person who battles to lose weight has slipped at least once . . . or twice, or many times. The secret is not to let a misstep become a landslide. Resist the urge to berate yourself or get discouraged and throw in the towel. Don't make more of the error than it deserves.

Start again—right away. Don't wait until the next day to get back on track. Remind yourself that the healthy weight-loss plan you have selected will work over time. Then learn from your mistake and move on. The only way to fail is to quit.

Don't let an occasional bad day
derail a lifetime of good health.

Lose Weight,

I Would . . .

Plan meals
in advance.

*Don't say you don't have enough
time. You have exactly the same
number of hours per day that were
given to Helen Keller, Louis
Pasteur, Michelangelo, Mother
Teresa, Leonardo DaVinci, Thomas
Jefferson, and Albert Einstein.*

—Unknown

Spur-of-the-moment meals generally mean fast food or deli takeout—both of which generally contain excess calories and fat grams. Plan meals in advance. Having a one-week plan helps in several ways: grocery shopping lists can be very specific, menus can be checked readily for nutritional balance, food treats can be sprinkled throughout the week to avert impulse binges, and the plan can serve as a checklist. Marking off items on such a list can be motivating.

As you plan menus, also plan your schedule to allow sufficient *time* both to prepare and consume nutritious meals. When planning to cook a special low-cal, low-fat dish, invite a friend to share the meal with you.

Most people don't plan to fail—
they simply fail to plan!

Lose Weight,

I Would . . .

Think about
what I eat.

Your thoughts become your words.
Your words become your actions.
Your actions become your habits.
Your habits become your character.
Your character becomes
your destiny.
—Unknown

We each have been given freedom of choice. Too often, however, we become creatures of habit and routine and lose sight of all the choices that we make, or *can* make, in a day.

Review and reevaluate your habits when it comes to eating and food. List habits in two columns—constructive and destructive. Then decide which habit you want to change *first* and plan an alternate course to take. Give yourself three weeks to make the change before tackling the next bad habit. Focus on where you are headed—toward more energy, greater fitness, and improved health—and not on what you have to give up to get there.

Conscious choices tend to be good choices.

Lose Weight,

I Would . . .

Stay on course when I hit a plateau.

❧

*Perseverance must finish
its work so that you may be
mature and complete, not
lacking anything.*
—James 1:4

Every person who embarks on a weight-loss program will hit at least one plateau—a time when the scale doesn't budge one pound, no matter what. How discouraging! There are several *good* reasons why this happens, however. The body periodically must adjust to weight loss. In some cases, fatty tissues are being converted to lean muscle weight. Weight can also fluctuate with water retention.

Plateaus can last a few days or even several weeks, but they can't defeat you if you stand firm and refuse to give up on your weight-loss goals. Focus on maintaining your healthy eating and exercise habits. Eventually, the scale will move again!

The goal is the process.

Lose Weight,

I Would . . .

Eat small meals often.

*Snacking is not the
problem of the American diet.
The snacks are the problem.
Preparation is the key to having
healthy snacks available.*
—David and Anne Frähm
Healthy Habits

Eating frequently is a good rule for several reasons: hunger is never allowed to build to the binge point, blood sugar levels are maintained at an even level (which eliminates hunger signals and produces a more steady level of energy), nutrition to the brain is more constant, and a person tends to think more clearly and make food decisions more rationally.

Many dietitians recommend five or six small meals a day, including afternoon and before-bedtime snacks and a mid-morning snack. Each meal should include protein since protein creates sustained energy over a longer period, and make sure that the total calorie and fat content of all the meals does not exceed your daily quota.

Eating smaller meals creates a pattern of eating less at each sitting.

Lose Weight,

I Would . . .

Identify my responses to stress.

I'm convinced that life is 10 percent what happens to me and 90 percent how I react to it.
—Charles R. Swindoll

For many people, anxiety triggers a desire for food. That's because eating soothes tension by releasing endorphins that encourage relaxation. However, there are other more productive ways to release those endorphins.

Exercise, for example, is an excellent way to relieve stress. Get on the treadmill, take a walk around the block, or get busy with some housework. Or, if you prefer, try the opposite approach—put on your favorite music, pour a cold glass of water with lemon, and take a hot sudsy bath. If you tend to "pig out" when you "stress out," build up your defenses by finding healthier alternatives to tension-induced uncontrolled eating.

Stressed is desserts spelled backwards!

Lose Weight,

I Would . . .

Avoid fad
diets.

*Do not be carried away by all
kinds of strange teachings.*
—Hebrews 13:9

Grapefruit . . . liquid protein . . . lettuce and cottage cheese . . . all fruit . . . all vegetables . . . no carbs . . . no sugar . . . no salt. What do all these diets have in common? No balance.

Fad diets work in the short term because they lower calorie intake. But over the long haul, they can deplete the body of vital nutrients and throw your system way out of balance. They become fad diets because they don't satisfy over time, and they are never a good way to keep the weight off. Choose instead to adopt a plan that can be used not only for weight loss but also as the foundation of a healthy lifestyle.

Taking care of yourself never goes out of style.

Use positive self-talk to reinforce my desired weight-loss plan and goals.

Whether you think you can or think you can't—you are right.
—Henry Ford

What are you telling yourself about you? What stream-of-consciousness tapes do you play in your head? Are you your own best friend or are you the devil's advocate? Each of us plays an interior tape of self-talk, speaking things to ourselves and about ourselves in our minds.

Self-talk is powerful because it is constant and intensely personal. It forms the base for what we believe about ourselves. Affirm yourself for achieving even small goals that help keep you on a long-term track toward good health and increased vitality. Reinforce the positive aspects of your own attitudes and behavior. Encourage yourself in your own quest for greater fitness. Become your own best cheerleader!

*Positive interior self-talk can lead
to positive external changes.*

Order an appetizer
for a main course
when dining out.

*Eat, drink, and be merry,
for tomorrow we shall diet.*
—Unknown

Eating out doesn't have to be a nightmare just because you are on a weight-loss program. There are many ways to enjoy your favorite restaurant without courting disaster.

Try a fresh salad bar, sticking to the greens and veggies and avoiding heavier pasta or potato salads. Or order a tasty, low fat appetizer as a main course. The serving portions are smaller, but usually adequate—in many cases, they are reduced-size portions of main dishes found elsewhere on the menu. You can also ask for a half portion or eat half and take the rest home with you. You'll be amazed how much better you will feel.

When dining out, think of every dish as "dinner for two"—either order half or take half home.

Lose Weight,

I Would . . .

Think in terms of health gain rather than weight loss.

If I had known I was going to live this long, I would have taken better care of myself.
—Unknown

Nobody likes to think in terms of losing. Think, instead, in terms of winning those things that make life more worthwhile—things like good health, more energy, and a better appearance, for starters.

People who are healthy and fit live longer and have a greater capacity for enjoying their lives. Losing weight means gaining strength and vitality, along with a more effective immune system. There's a great deal to be *gained* by losing unwanted pounds. In the end, you will gain an increased ability to be all that you can be.

❧

Your loss can also be your gain.

Lose Weight,

I Would . . .

Weigh regularly.

❦

When I saw it, I considered it well; I looked on it and received instruction.
—Proverbs 24:32 NKJV

Some people find it helpful to weigh daily—sort of an early-morning reality check. Others recommend a weekly weigh-in, at the same time each week, since weight can fluctuate a pound or two daily depending on fluid retention.

Regardless of how frequently you weigh, discipline yourself to weigh regularly on a reliable scale. Keep track of your progress, and focus on the number you *want* to see on the scale. Remember, too, that the scale isn't the only measure of success. If you are exercising and turning fat to muscle, you may not see much change on the scale. Pay attention to the way your clothes fit in conjunction with weight loss.

"Ignore it and it will go away"
does not apply to excess weight.

Lose Weight,

I Would . . .

Refuse to deprive myself of all my favorite foods.

There is nothing to be ashamed of in enjoying your food: there would be everything to be ashamed of if half the world made food the main intent of their lives. . . .

—C. S. Lewis

It's easy to feel deprived when your friends are packing away the pizza, cheeseburgers, and fries while you stick to the salad bar. That's why a weight-loss program that deprives you of all your favorite foods will not succeed. What can you do?

Make wise compromises; an effective weight-loss plan is not *all* of one type of food and *none* of the other. Try sharing that cheeseburger with someone, and exchange the fries for a small salad or a scoop of cottage cheese and a pineapple slice. Enjoy the half of the cheeseburger you are eating, rather than bemoan the half you aren't eating. You *can* enjoy all foods . . . just not all at once!

There is no forbidden food, just problem foods in problem quantities.

Lose Weight,

I Would . . .

Exercise after work and before eating dinner.

Everyone who competes in the games goes into strict training.
—1 Corinthians 9:25

The hour just after work or school is the time when most people feel the least energetic, and it is also the time when people are likely to grab a high-calorie snack to recharge. Rather than stopping at a fast-food place on your way home from work, try a workout instead.

Early-day exercise boosts metabolism, and late-afternoon exercise both vents stress and keeps the metabolism running at peak into the evening hours. A late-afternoon workout will actually reduce your appetite for dinner and replenish your energy for the evening. Plus, it helps you relax and sleep better.

Turn the "happy hour" into a fitness hour—you'll be more than happy with the results!

Lose Weight,

I Would . . .

Leave off
the sauces.

*The good news is that flavorful,
lower-fat cooking is easier than
I thought . . . best of all–
the clean, clear fresh tastes
are memorable, satisfying, and
easy to trust every day.*
—Julee Rosso

Great Good Food

Think of sauces, gravies, toppings, grated cheese, and dressings as globs of fat that are put over otherwise nutritious foods. In many cases, they are precisely that. A baked potato, for example, has relatively few calories and high fiber content. Add rich toppings, however, and the calorie count can soar. A piece of grilled, skinned chicken has relatively few calories and is a good source of protein—add gravy or sauces and all the benefits can be negated.

Choose to eat foods plain, or season dishes with fresh herbs and spices that add flavor and variety without adding calories. If you must add a topping, choose a no-fat version.

Leave the spoons in the drawer. What you don't spoon over food doesn't add weight!

Refuse to let a bad day become an excuse to quit.

*I am not concerned that
you have fallen—I am
concerned that you arise.*
—Abraham Lincoln

Countless books exist about how to succeed. But the secret to success seems to come down to one single point: the successful person gets up one more time than he falls down. If you have had a bad day, don't give up. Concentrate on identifying and changing the root causes that compelled you to err.

You might also try scheduling break days into your weight-loss program—days when you allow yourself to eat larger portions or to eat foods that are normally not on your plan. Develop a "Plan B" for getting back on course when you have a bad day.

Lapses are inevitable . . . but recovery is always possible!

I Would . . .

Solicit the support of friends.

We . . . sent Timothy, our brother and minister of God . . . to establish you and encourage you.
—1 Thessalonians 3:1,2 NKJV

There's nothing like talking, or listening, to someone who is living a parallel experience. That's why support groups are so helpful to a successful weight-loss plan. Not only can you motivate and encourage one another, but you can share helpful tips and low-fat, low-calorie recipes and cooking ideas.

Ask your friends to help you by *not* talking about food in your presence—including talk about new restaurants they have tried or new dishes they have prepared. They can also help by *not* asking you to try "just one bite" of their dessert. If a person becomes a routine tempter, avoid that person until you have reached your goal.

❦

Good friends want what is best for each other.

Lose Weight,

I Would . . .

Cut the size of serving portions.

❧

Take nothing in excess.
—Socrates

Cut serving sizes of calorie-rich foods in half, or at least by one-third, and you have reduced a significant number of calories! Rather than putting two slices of cheese on a sandwich, use one. Rather than having a half-pound hamburger patty, have a quarter-pounder. Take one scoop of casserole instead of two. Then fill up the extra space on the plate with salad or steamed vegetables. Use smaller serving utensils to serve food.

As you begin to cut portions, you'll be surprised at how satisfied you are with the smaller serving. You'll save fat, calories, and that uncomfortable, discouraging feeling that accompanies overeating.

Portion patrol your plate!

Lose Weight,

I Would . . .

Try new recipes that are low-cal and low-fat, but tasty!

*Good taste is essential
to food enjoyment.*
—Graham Kerr
Minimax Cookbook

Preparing food that *tastes* good is essential to the success of any weight-loss program. Fortunately, in recent years, nutritionists have responded to the demand for healthful, weight-related products by developing countless *tasty* low-calorie, low-fat recipes. And these recipes are almost always surprisingly easy to prepare.

Alternate spices, seasonings, and low-fat marinades pack all the taste without the fat. In fact, sugar and fat often mask the true taste of foods. Most people discover that if they give low-fat food a fair try, they develop a preference for it over time. Rediscover how good food can taste in its natural state!

Eating right whets your appetite for healthy food.

Lose Weight,

I Would . . .

Adopt new cooking techniques that are more healthful.

*Say to him: "Long life to you!
Good health to you and your
household! And good health
to all that is yours!"*
—1 Samuel 25:6

Like fried foods? Forget the breading and try stir-frying instead. An atomizer is a good way to spray oil on a pan or wok, or you can use an unsaturated cooking spray. Be adventurous with herbs, fresh garlic and ginger, veggies, and lean meats. Cooking with a wok does not need to mean Oriental fare.

For great French fries, spray a cookie sheet with oil and cover it with thin slices or sticks of fresh potatoes. Or roast lean meats and vegetables in foil cooking bags—either in the oven or on the grill. Look for low-fat recipes that you can enjoy for years to come—not just while you are losing weight.

Changing cooking styles can open up a whole new world of taste!

Lose Weight,

I Would . . .

Drink more water.

Open his eyes, shut off by clouds
From the thousand fountains
So near him, dying of thirst
In his own desert.
                    —Goethe

Medical researchers have discovered that water may be the single most important catalyst in losing weight and keeping it off. Water is a natural appetite suppresser and actually helps the body metabolize stored fat.

Studies show that a decrease in water intake causes fat deposits to increase, while an increase in water intake can actually reduce fat deposits. In addition, water helps the body to flush away undesirable toxins and fatty globules from the blood stream. It is a major aid to maintaining good digestion and elimination. On the average, a person should drink eight glasses of water every day. An overweight person should add to that an extra glass for every twenty-five pounds of excess weight.

Water is a natural enemy of fat.

If I Really
Wanted to

Lose Weight,

I Would . . .

Fire up
the grill.

Grilled Salmon

2–3 salmon steaks, 2 garlic cloves, pressed,
2 teaspoons fresh lemon zest,
2–3 teaspoons fresh lemon juice, salt and
pepper for seasoning.
Combine ingredients, rub on steaks, and
grill. . . .

—Kristine Fortier

Recipes for Healthy Living

With so many wonderful, low-fat seasonings and marinades, you'll want to grill nearly everything! It is a good way to add flavor to meats and vegetables, especially as you experiment with different types of wood chips. More flavor for vegetables can result in more vegetables being consumed!

Those who don't particularly enjoy cooking or eating fish often find that grilling makes *eating* fish far more satisfying—and cooking outdoors eliminates cooking odors. Outdoor grilling has one added benefit: others can nearly always be coaxed into helping with the cooking, and that will help you avoid nibbling as you work.

Lighting the grill is a good way to "lite" up a weight-loss plan.

Lose Weight,

I Would . . .

Work with a physician to establish and track my weight loss goals.

❧

Plans fail for lack of counsel, but with many advisors they succeed.
—Proverbs 15:22

Your physician is one of the best allies you can have when you are following a weight-loss plan. Most appreciate having the opportunity to be on the preventive side of medicine and enjoy sharing tips. Let your physician help you establish incremental goals and an exercise plan that is safe for you. In most cases, he or she will even help you develop a personalized plan if you ask.

Take advantage of the resources already available to you by involving your physician in whatever plan you have chosen. You will find that the advice, encouragement, and peace of mind are well worth it.

Lose weight, but keep your health.

Lose Weight,

I Would . . .

Not eat on the run or while in my car.

You are where you eat.
—Unknown

Do you find yourself picking up a snack here or a burger there because you're pressed for time? Unfortunately, you may be paying a higher price for convenience than you imagine.

Realistically, your options for healthier fare are slim to none in a fast food restaurant. Going home and sitting down to eat will help you eat slower. Light some candles, turn off the television, and put on some music. Make mealtime an experience that satisfies the eyes, ears, *and* taste buds. You will feed both body and soul—and many times, the more adequately the soul is fed, the less food the body seems to require.

Feed your soul as well as your body.

Lose Weight,

I Would . . .

Avoid alcohol
(and other high-sugar drinks).

[Alcohol] is worse than useless. It not only fails to add to daily nutritional requirements, but actually interferes with good eating habits and with the body's ability to use the nutrients in the other foods that we consume.

—Allan Luks and Joseph Barbato

You Are What You Drink

Alcohol can defeat your weight-loss plan in two key ways. One, alcohol stimulates the appetite—not the best idea when your goal is to lose weight. In addition, alcoholic beverages, and especially mixed drinks, are high in sugar and thus, high in calories.

A far better approach is to drink herb teas or pure water. Also avoid non-alcoholic beverages that can be high in sugar—including most fruit drinks, sweetened teas, and most flavored waters. Even sparkling water and carbonated beverages should be curtailed in number since they tend to have high-sodium counts, which can cause fluid retention. Retained fluids show up as pounds, which can result in discouragement.

Make water or herb tea your beverage of choice.

Lose Weight,

I Would . . .

Clean out my kitchen cupboards.

*If your eye causes you
to sin, gouge it out and
throw it away.*
—Matthew 18:9

If having fattening foods in your cupboards is a temptation, by all means, get rid of them! "Out of sight, out of mind" is a good rule to follow. If you don't have fattening foods in your cupboards—or refrigerator, freezer, or pantry—you will not be able to put your hands on them when hunger strikes and resolve melts away.

Instead, stock your cupboard and refrigerator shelves with healthful fruits and vegetables, which are more compatible for long-term weight loss. Such snacking can actually stimulate your metabolism and contribute to your efforts. You are not only altering what you eat but also how you approach eating.

To focus on what is positive and healthful, eliminate what is tempting and non-productive.

Keep a
food diary.

The bearings of this observation
lays in the application on it.
—Charles Dickens

A food diary can be of great help as you lose weight and change the way you eat. Write down *every bite* you put into your mouth, including gum and breath mints. The diary will point out the little slips that add up to seriously sabotage your weight-loss plan.

Also record the calorie and fat content of the foods you eat. This will help you learn which meals satisfy with the least cost to your plan. Increase your water consumption each week for several weeks and track that too. Make notes about your attitude and energy level at each meal. And be sure you look back and apply the knowledge you get from the information you've recorded.

Keeping an honest food diary is
a way of learning about yourself.

Lose Weight,

I Would . . .

Reduce my
red-meat intake.

*All the nutritional requirements that the
human body has—all the vitamins,
minerals, proteins, amino acids, enzymes,
carbohydrates, and fatty acids that exist,
that the human body needs to survive—
are to be found in fruits and vegetables.*
—Harvey and Marilyn Diamond
Fit for Life

This is not to suggest that you become a vegetarian, but lessening your red-meat intake can be helpful. While red meat is a good source of protein, it also tends to be high in fat and calories.

Eat beef, pork, and lamb only once or twice a week, and add more poultry and fish to your menu. Also experiment with other sources of protein that are low in fat, such as tofu, soy milk, nonfat dairy products, protein powders, eggs (especially no-cholesterol egg products), and legumes. When you do have that special occasion steak, remove all the fat possible. Also remove the skin before eating chicken. Grill, broil, or roast meats, rather than frying or sautéing them.

Less red meat . . . fewer calories.

Lose Weight,

I Would . . .

Say no to second helpings.

*Like a city whose walls are
broken down is a man
who lacks self-control.*
—Proverbs 25:28

When former First Lady Nancy Reagan initially proposed that people "just say no" to an offer of drugs, many people laughed, "If only life could be that simple!" they protested. However, in many cases, just saying no is the best approach a person can take, and especially when it comes to food intake.

When someone says "How about a second helping?" they may not realize it, but they are actually saying, "Here, have a double portion of calories and fat grams." Just smile and say, "No! Thank you very much." And as they tell school children in every anti-drug program, every time you say "no," the next time is a little easier.

❧

You need say no more than to say "no more."

Lose Weight,

I Would . . .

Combine watching TV with exercise.

Dost thou love life? Then do not squander time; for that's the stuff life is made of.
—Benjamin Franklin

If you have half an hour to watch television, you also have a half hour for exercise! Walk on a treadmill, ride an exercise bike, or use other exercise equipment. And, if television isn't your choice of entertainment, there are plenty of other things you can do.

Try listening to motivational audio tapes, watching instructional or inspirational videos, or listening to books on tape. You might enjoy taping a program while you are at work and watching it while you exercise. If walking or riding in place isn't fun for you, add some entertainment to make the activity more pleasant. Make the most of every moment of every day—you'll never get it back!

Rather than being a couch potato, choose to be an active viewer.

Lose Weight,

I Would . . .

Get sufficient nutrients.

*For decades people have believed
that eating a balanced diet
provided all the nutrients they
needed. It's simply not true.*
—Michael Janson, M.D.

Health and Nutrition Breakthroughs
March 1998

Food cravings can be a signal that key nutrients are missing from your diet or that they are not being supplied in adequate amounts. Unfortunately, we often seek to satisfy cravings with foods that are high in calories, sugars, and fat. What many dieters don't know is that cravings for wrong foods—such as chocolate and sugary foods—can actually be eliminated over time by eating foods higher in protein.

To make certain that you receive all of the micro-nutrients your body needs in adequate quantities, consider adding vitamins, minerals, and protein supplements to your weight-loss plan. Work with a nutritionist to determine the best options or simply ask your physician or pharmacist.

Feed your cells all of the nutrients they need.

Lose Weight,

I Would . . .

Refuse to be tricked by claims that make food products appear healthier.

The wise man has eyes in his head, while the fool walks in the darkness.

—Ecclesiastes 2:14

Be a discerning consumer. A chocolate product recently was labeled "no cholesterol." True enough—but nothing about the product's sugar content or calorie count had been altered. "No cholesterol" in this case still meant high-calorie, and excess calories are stored as fat.

Keep in mind always that low-fat is not the same as nonfat or no-fat. "Reduced calories" is not the same as low in calories, and "low-calorie" must always be considered a relative term. "No sugar" does not mean no fat, and "no-fat" does not mean no-calorie. Check the labels for actual calories and grams of fat. And when faced with products that claim to be healthy, low, "lite," or reduced, always ask, "compared to what?"

❧

An "almost free ride" is still going to cost you something.

If I Really
Wanted to

Lose Weight,

I Would . . .

Eat larger meals earlier rather than later in the day.

Man is not the creature of circumstances. Circumstances are the creatures of men.
—Benjamin Disraeli

Metabolism is the rate at which your body burns calories, converting food into energy. This rate varies from person to person and fluctuates throughout the day. In the morning, your metabolism starts off slow, but gradually picks up speed throughout the day. Then it drops to its lowest level at night. Exercising early boosts your metabolism to pick up speed earlier in the day, giving your body a greater opportunity to burn off the calories rather than store them as fat.

The bottom line is that the earlier in the day you eat your meals, the better your body will burn off the calories you consume. Take control of your circumstances, and eat to lose and to maintain your ideal weight.

*Work with your own body rhythms,
not against them!*

If I Really
Wanted to
Lose Weight,
I Would . . .

Invest in a good low-cal, low-fat cookbook.

We are realizing that what we have thought of as standard fare can be exciting and inventive. Try Poppy Seed Pasta, Mexican Kasha or Southwestern Black-eyed Peas. . . .
—Betty Crocker's 40th Anniversary Edition Cookbook

Part of retraining yourself for healthy weight loss and maintenance includes knowing how to prepare foods that are not only good for you, but also taste good. Even standard cookbooks are seeing the value of nutritious, low fat, inventive cooking, especially for busy lifestyles. A good low-calorie, low-fat cookbook can offer lots of tips for dishes that *don't* taste like cardboard and are genuinely satisfying.

Experiment with new recipes. And if possible, find a book that offers tips for substituting low-cal, low-fat ingredients for more fattening ingredients in traditional recipes. Consider a good healthy-eating cookbook as a sound investment for many years to come.

Good recipes can still translate into good news for weight loss.

Lose Weight,

I Would . . .

Become "gram" conscious.

*Every prudent man acts
out of knowledge.*
—Proverbs 13:16

Think about getting yourself a small scale and a couple of good, portable nutrition books. Look up the calorie, cholesterol, or fat-gram content of foods that you are preparing to eat—you may be surprised at what you discover.

Weigh foods so that you become better informed about what a four-ounce chicken breast *looks* like compared to a six-ounce chicken breast. Then look up the difference between skinned and skinless and between a chicken breast and a chicken thigh and leg. The more you are able to determine *by sight* the nutritional value of food items, the better you will be able to control your weight over time.

Knowing how much of a good thing to eat is important.

Lose Weight,

I Would . . .

Steam or broil food to save calories and retain flavor.

❧

Appetite comes with eating.
—French Proverb

Broiling, poaching, and steaming require little or no added oil. These methods do not add extra calories to a meal, and they can actually reduce the calories in many traditional recipes.

When you steam vegetables, for example, they retain their flavor and nutrients rather than losing them in the cooking water. In-pot steamers are inexpensive. Vertical roasters ensure that chickens and turkeys do not cook while setting in their own fat. And don't forget to look for the words "broiled" and "steamed" on menus when dining out. Pretty soon, your palate will tell you to stick with the essence of wonderful, fresh foods.

Gain food flavor from freshness, not fat!

Lose Weight,

I Would . . .

Think green
and leafy.

*Never eat more
than you can lift.*
—Miss Piggy

Not only are they light and genteel, but they offer much more substantial benefit. Green and leafy vegetables tend to give more nutrient value per calorie than most other foods. They provide good fiber and bulk to help you feel full faster. Some greens, such as broccoli, are known to contain nutrients that can help protect against auto-immune diseases such as cancer.

Fresh leafy vegetables are not just for salads—some heartier greens such as bok choy are terrific when braised or used in stir-fry. Most of these vegetables have a negative calorie count, which means they require the body to burn more calories to digest them than the vegetables have. What a deal!

Eat all you want of green and leafy vegetables.

Lose Weight,

I Would . . .

Set a training goal.

❧

Therefore, I do not run like a man running aimlessly; I do not fight like a man beating the air.
—1 Corinthians 9:26

A woman with muscular dystrophy spent years saying "I can't" to things she wanted to do. One day she decided to set a goal to run the New York City marathon. Much to the surprise of many, she finished the race and accomplished her goal! It was painful for her to prepare for the race and painful to run it, but she later told the world that every step was worth the pain.

To keep yourself motivated in an exercise program, set a training goal—perhaps to walk a mile in eight minutes, row across a local lake, hike a certain trail, or swim a half mile. Set incremental goals for achieving your final training goal. Then focus and begin "the race."

Every hour of activity is an hour of calorie expenditure.

Lose Weight,

I Would . . .

Try a new physical challenge.

*You've got to continue to grow,
or you're like last night's
cornbread—stale and dry.*
—Loretta Lynn

Experts say if a person sticks with an exercise routine for thirty days, it becomes a habit. Yet even good habits can get boring. To keep your exercise regimen interesting, try a new activity that sounds interesting to you. Choose one with which you are unfamiliar so that it requires your total concentration and motivates you to keep learning—perhaps something such as para-sailing, inline skating, square dancing, water ballet, beach volleyball, or water polo.

You don't have to become a master at the new sport—you simply have to like it enough, and be challenged enough by it, to keep yourself moving. Inevitably, you'll grow as a person in the process.

Rediscover how much fun active play can be!

Lose Weight,

I Would . . .

Put an inspiring photo on the refrigerator door.

A rock pile ceases to be a rock pile the moment a single man contemplates it, bearing within him the image of a cathedral.
—Antoine de Saint-Exupéry

Develop the habit of focusing your inner vision less on the foods you shouldn't eat and more on something that, for you, will make weight loss truly worthwhile.

Put photos on your refrigerator door— perhaps a photo of a place you plan to go when you reach your goal or a photo of the way you looked before you gained weight. Consider posting a photo of the family that would appreciate a more energetic and healthier you or some other reason that you have for getting more fit, such as a photo of a mountain you hope to climb one day. Maybe you would find the words of your favorite saying or Scripture more inspiring. Either way—hold that thought!

Positive thoughts lead to positive actions.

Lose Weight,

I Would . . .

Shop for groceries on a full stomach.

❧

*Once when Jacob was cooking some
stew, Esau came in from the open
country, famished. He said to Jacob,
"Quick, let me have some of that red
stew! I'm famished!" . . . Jacob
replied, "First sell me your birthright."
"Look, I am about to die," Esau said.
"What good is the birthright to me?"*
—Genesis 25:29–32

While a bad shopping trip doesn't exactly equal the gravity of giving up one's birthright, it can cause you to jump the track on the way to your weight-loss destination. Even if you make and stick to a strict shopping list, foods that normally wouldn't appeal to you become nearly irresistible when you're hungry. Add the temptation of free food samples in every other aisle and abundant aromas from the deli.

Shopping on a full stomach is much less likely to leave you feeling either tempted or deprived. If you can't shop right *after* eating, drink a large glass of water before entering a grocery store.

⁂

*Shopping on a full stomach
helps you avoid obstacles.*

Lose Weight,

I Would . . .

Keep fruits and vegetables washed, cut up, and ready to eat in the refrigerator.

*There is more acknowledgment by
men of science that raw, uncooked food
in the diet is indispensable to the
highest degree of health.*

—Richard O. Brennan, D.O., M.D.

Coronary? Cancer? God's Answer: Prevent It!

One of the best—and easiest—ways to gain control of weight is to keep the refrigerator stocked with fruits and vegetables that are cleaned, chopped up, and ready to eat. This ensures that good, low fat, low calorie foods are available for after-work, after-school, and after-dinner snacks.

Having veggies cut up and ready to go also makes salad preparation and sack-lunch preparation quicker and easier—which means you are more likely to make and *eat* a salad or to take nutritious foods to work or school for the noon meal. Don't wait until you're hungry and willpower is ebbing—set the stage for success.

Make it easy to make the right choices!

Lose Weight,

I Would . . .

Choose to eat more fresh and whole foods.

*Knowest thou the land
where the lemon-trees bloom,
Where the gold orange
glows in the deep thicket's gloom,
Where a wind ever soft
from the blue heaven blows,
And the groves are of laurel
and myrtle and rose?*

—Goethe

While the majority of us don't have access to plentiful, poetry-inspiring orchards, we can get whole, fresh foods, the taste of which should inspire us to enjoy them every day. These foods offer greater taste variety and potency, which means that smaller quantities offer more satisfaction.

Whole, fresh foods also tend to be lower in calorie, sodium and fat content, since hydrogenated oils and sugars are often added during processing. Plus, fresh foods add the right kinds of fiber to the diet. Most vegetables and many fruits are lower in per-serving sugars and calories than baked, fried, or packaged foods. When you eat whole and fresh foods, you get more nutrition and taste per bite!

Whole and fresh foods stimulate the palate.

Lose Weight,

I Would . . .

Remind my family that encouragement is a big help during a weight-loss program.

A word aptly spoken is like apples of gold in settings of silver.
—Proverbs 25:11

Before you begin your weight-loss program, talk to your family and tell them you need their prayers, encouragement, and understanding as you undertake a change in the way you are eating. Explain that you need cheers, not jeers, to get you back on track when you slip. Ask them not to tempt you to eat foods that are not a part of your weight-loss plan.

As time passes, let them know you've done well so they can celebrate with you. Thank them for helping you with supportive words and actions. And for heaven's sake, receive their compliments, even if you're not as far along as you'd like to be in your plan.

Enlist your family members as your cheerleaders.

Lose Weight,

I Would . . .

When dining out, always ask for salad dressing and condiments on the side.

*God helps them that
help themselves.*
—Ben Franklin

When you choose to eat out, you voluntarily give up a certain amount of control over the calorie content of the foods you order. But many restaurants seem to go overboard on the quantity of sauces, condiments, and dressings they put on various dishes. You can take back control over the calories in these items by asking that they be served on the side.

Add salad dressing a little at a time so you only consume what is necessary. Use sauces and other condiments as dips for each bite. Always try a food item dry before doctoring it with extras. You may decide you prefer the taste of the food in its pure state.

*When you eat away from home,
take your common sense with you.*

Lose Weight,

I Would . . .

Read the labels on food products.

❧

*Problems cannot be solved
at the same level of awareness
that created them.*
—Albert Einstein

Read the nutrition labels on products to find out what percentage of the total calorie count is fat, and don't be fooled by the words "lite," "low fat," or "reduced fat." They may simply mean that the product contains *less* fat than the regular version of the same product. Mayonnaise, for example, is nearly all fat, and low-fat mayonnaise is still mostly fat! To lose weight, a person must keep fat intake at five to ten percent of the total calories consumed.

Beware, too, of products that may be low in fat but high in sugar. Sugar and carbohydrates are also stored as fat!

Believe the nutrition label more than the front label on food products.

Lose Weight,

I Would . . .

Thank God for all signs of progress.

Praise be to the LORD, to God our Savior, who daily bears our burdens.
—Psalm 68:19

Go into a weight-loss program with one key word in mind—patience. The first week is usually the most difficult and often can pass without many signs of progress. Even so, thank God that you are conquering food challenges and changing habits every day. Keep a log of weight and size losses with space for writing prayers, comments, and observations. Use weight-loss days as opportunities for thanks and praise.

When your weight stays the same for days, ask God for renewed strength to withstand temptation . . . and then, continue to offer praise that God is with you always. In doing this, your spirit will grow as your body decreases.

❧

It's difficult to lose your footing
when you're on your knees.

Lose Weight,

I Would . . .

Decide before entering a restaurant what I want to order.

❧

Where you eat determines what you eat. Choose restaurants that serve the healthy foods you want. Go there more often.

—Mayo Clinic

Eating Well When Eating Out

The first ten minutes in a restaurant are the most treacherous. Already hungry, you are bombarded by smells and visual images of food being eaten by others nearby. And then the menu arrives and every item described seems irresistible.

Generally decide what you are going to order several hours before you arrive at the restaurant and have a backup item in mind in case your first choice is unavailable. Check the menu only to confirm that your choice is available and then place it out of reach. Do the same with table cards describing special desserts or food items.

Don't play with fire by lingering over a menu.

Lose Weight,

I Would . . .

Split the

dessert.

*Small amounts of food can
lead to consumption of fewer
calories, less expense, and
permanent weight loss.*
—Graham Kerr

Minimax Cookbook

Occasional indulgences—especially if they are planned and part of a good long-term plan—can actually contribute to the success of your weight-loss plan. *Always* skipping dessert is no way to live, and therefore, it is no way to lose weight. Two tips, however, can cut the calorie intake of a dessert.

Either split the dessert with a dining companion or ask for a take-home container when you order. Put half of the dessert in the container and close it before you begin eating the rest. Either give the take-home half to a family member or plan for the extra calories as part of a menu later in the week.

You CAN enjoy goodies and build good habits at the same time.

Lose Weight,

I Would . . .

Never eat food from its original container.

*Let all things be done
decently and in order.*
—1 Corinthians 14:40 KJV

Always place food onto a plate or bowl before eating it; and always pour beverages into drinking glasses. This applies even to so-called "individual serving size" containers. And try never to eat standing up; always find a place to sit down and place the food on a table in front of you.

In establishing these patterns, you are exerting control over the food items you consume and creating a meal with thoughtful planning. You are likely to prepare more balanced meals, with each item in proper quantity. Subconsciously, you're more apt to realize you've eaten if you make it a conscious affair.

Treat yourself with dignity at each meal.

Lose Weight,

I Would . . .

Not skip breakfast or any other meal.

Breakfast is the most important meal of the day.
—Your Mother

As you lose weight, you want your body to burn excess stored fat efficiently without burning lean muscle tissue. But when you skip a meal, your body naturally goes into a preservation mode. The brain signals your metabolism to slow down so your body can survive on its current storehouse of calories for as long as possible. Energy used for vital bodily functions is pulled from stored fat but *also* from lean muscle tissue—including the heart muscle.

That's a dangerous trend over time! Regular eating keeps your metabolism running at peak levels and encourages your body to use both the new intake of food for energy as well as the stored fat, without pulling nutrients from muscle.

Give your body what it needs to run efficiently and burn fat.

Lose Weight,

I Would . . .

Stay away from the donut box at work.

*Take away the brakes and
your life, like your car, is
transformed into an unguided
missile—destined for disaster.*
—Charles R. Swindoll

An old television commercial proclaimed with gusto, "Time to make the donuts!" While there is nothing wrong with donut *making,* many people have adopted a slightly different version as a routine morning slogan, "Time to eat the donuts!" Stop to consider how many miles a person needs to walk to work off the calories in just one glazed donut. The answer is "more miles than most people are willing to walk!"

The donut box, the dessert trolley, the lidded cake plate, and the food sections of most quick-stop stores and gas-station markets are places that you should avoid if you want to lose weight successfully.

Could it be that Pandora's box contained a mixed dozen?

Lose Weight,

I Would . . .

Refuse to take diet pills.

*Do you not know that your body
is a temple of the Holy Spirit,
who is in you, whom you
have received from God?*
—1 Corinthians 6:19

Please, please, please—do not take diet pills. They, along with various other diet products, have far more potential for harm than for good. What good is a skinny body if your organs or body systems are damaged?

Furthermore, the person who relies upon a pill or potion is likely avoiding the real issues associated with weight management and health—a need for information about good nutrition, to make wiser choices, or to exert willpower. Good results can always be achieved *without* pills and potions. It's also important to note that tobacco products should never be used as weight-loss aids—they always produce more harm than benefit to the body.

❧

Develop a plan for losing weight that does not sabotage your future health.

Lose Weight,

I Would . . .

Drink a glass of water before each meal.

Water, water everywhere,
Nor any drop to drink.
—Samuel Taylor Coleridge

Drinking a glass of water before eating means less food is needed in order for you to feel full. Water is also a natural diuretic—an intake of water tells the brain that it is going to receive adequate fluid and therefore, less existing water needs to be retained in the body.

Water has no calories—but drinking very cold water can actually cause calories to be burned, since the body must work to raise the temperature of the water to body temperature. If you don't enjoy drinking water, add a slice of lemon or lime, or add a few drops of flavoring extract to an entire pitcher of water and use it to make ice cubes.

Make a glass of water the first course of every meal.

Lose Weight,

I Would . . .

Eat a sufficient amount of fiber.

&

*A high-fiber diet can help lower
cholesterol and may protect you
from colon problems... [and]
reduce your risk for diabetes.*
—Mayo Clinic Health Letter
March 1998

Fiber is your weight-loss friend. It fills your stomach quicker than fats and proteins and generally keeps the digestive tract in good running order. And it is not absorbed by the body, which is what makes it good roughage. But fiber has another very useful property. To varying degrees depending on the specific source, fiber tends to attract and bind to fat. It thus helps fat move through and out the digestive tract without being absorbed or stored in the body.

Fibrous vegetables and many grains and seeds are high in fiber content. Check a nutrition book to learn which items are recommended most by physicians.

High fiber is an important clue in a low-fat quest.

Lose Weight,

I Would . . .

Invest in a good scale.

*Use honest scales and
honest weights.*
—Leviticus 19:36

We hear, "To thine own self be true" in Shakespeare's *Hamlet,* and that's no less true when it comes to your weight-loss plan. Eliminate the guesswork and the all-too-familiar excuse of "the scale weighs heavy." Get out of denial and into reality. Tell yourself the truth about your weight and the potential consequences for your health and well-being.

This does not mean that you should beat up on yourself or hold yourself in contempt. It does mean that you need to look squarely at the truth, accept it as truth, and then act on the truth in a positive way. Honesty about weight is *always* the best policy.

✧

Denial weighs heavily on more than just the mind.

Lose Weight,

I Would . . .

Consider the big picture.

Nothing can stop the man with the right mental attitude from achieving his goal; nothing on earth can help the man with the wrong mental attitude.
—Thomas Jefferson

A recent study found that far more individuals maintain their weight loss over the long term than previously believed. The main reasons cited for this success were changes in eating and exercise habits. New, healthful habits had replaced the old ones that led to excess weight gain. Always choose a weight-loss plan with the big picture in mind—choose a plan that will help you develop the habits that can lead to healthful, nutritious eating three, six, and even ten years from now.

A long-range focus can also help you overcome discouragement about short-term plateaus and take away the feeling of deprivation. Keep a far-reaching perspective, and soon it will become an intrinsic part of your thought process.

Get through each day by keeping a future-oriented perspective.

Lose Weight,

I Would . . .

Learn to appreciate the way God made me.

*I praise you, for I am fearfully
and wonderfully made.
Wonderful are your works;
that I know very well.*
—Psalm 139:14 NRSV

From billboards and television commercials to magazine layouts, we are bombarded with images of the modern ideal of beauty. If those images become your goal, your weight-loss plan is likely to be doomed.

Don't seek to be like someone else or live up to another person's idea about how you should look. Begin to appreciate the body you were given by your Creator. You are a unique individual in every way, with priceless spiritual, mental, and physical characteristics. In God's eyes, you are beautiful and beloved, regardless of how much you weigh.

You are God's treasured work of art because you're a one-of-a-kind, made in the image of the most beautiful, supreme Being—our living God.

Lose Weight,

I Would . . .

Get in touch
with my body.

❧

Know thyself.
—Socrates

Learn to distinguish genuine physical hunger from other needs that are often disguised as hunger. Real hunger originates in an empty stomach and is accompanied by a lack of energy and ability to concentrate. Signals we often mistake for hunger are boredom; a need for a break, stretch, or exercise; stress; and the need for comfort.

When you *think* you need food, ask yourself if you are truly hungry physically or if you are really in need of something else— perhaps a chat with a friend, a brisk walk, or a break for fun. And don't be afraid to feel hungry. Experience it. Then you'll be sure to know your body's hunger signal.

Don't use food as a boredom breaker or incentive reward.

Lose Weight,

I Would . . .

Use substitutes for fat and sugar when cooking and baking.

৵৵

While it sometimes seems that no nutritional recommendation is valid for more than a few months, the need to significantly reduce total fat intake is a consistent message from the experts.

—Julee Rosso

Great Good Food

Thankfully, deprivation and sacrifice are words of the past. Today's words are substitution and modification. You don't have to sacrifice taste to eat healthfully. Try reducing the amount of sugar by one-half in many standard dessert recipes. Instead of putting butter on vegetables, add flavor by using spices, herbs, and flavored vinegars. Substitute ground turkey for ground beef. Use mustard instead of mayonnaise. Lower-calorie cocoa powder can be substituted for chocolate. Substitute nonfat yogurt for sour cream; use skim milk. Substitute chicken bouillon for butter in making mashed potatoes.

The list of healthful substitutions is endless. You can find an abundant number of resources for low-fat cooking and baking in books and online—start experimenting!

❧

Permanent weight loss requires permanent changes in eating and cooking habits.

If I Really
Wanted to

Lose Weight,

I Would . . .

Reserve some foods for celebrations.

*And bring the fatted calf
here and kill it, and
let us eat and be merry.*
—Luke 15:23 NKJV

Don't join in the lament, "I'll never be able to eat the foods I enjoy again." This statement is simply not true. More likely to be true is the statement, "I will need to eat the foods I love less often and in smaller quantities." Reserve some of your favorite recipes for special celebration times. Other foods might be factored into your menu plan once a month. Still other foods might be enjoyed on a smaller scale. Rather than indulging in an ice-cream sundae, for example, choose one scoop of ice cream.

Total deprivation can be demoralizing and is never required for weight loss or good weight management. Disciplining yourself as to quantity and frequency *are* required.

Discipline allows you to avoid deprivation.

Lose Weight,

I Would . . .

Eat with others and spend more time conversing than chewing.

Delicious. Isn't that an attractive word? It sums up so many joyful memories, not just of food, but people and places.

—Graham Kerr

Minimax Cookbook

Mother's advice to keep quiet and eat your dinner may have been necessary when you were a child, but now that you are an adult, you'll likely find it far more advantageous to eat less and talk more. If the mouth is busy holding up one end of a conversation, the food on the plate will have a more difficult time making it to the palate.

Pause periodically in your conversation to evaluate whether you are genuinely full. Eat enough to assuage genuine hunger, but then push away your plate and focus solely on the person sitting opposite you. Good conversation is satisfying, and it has no calories!

Make your meals a conversational experience you can remember with fondness!

Lose Weight,

I Would . . .

Tend a garden.

Vegetable gardening is for the adventuresome, imaginative child in each of us.
It's never dull.
—Suzanne Frutig Bales
American Gardening Series

Tending a garden provides two great bonuses for your weight-loss plan. First, pulling weeds, hoeing, shoveling, tilling, and pruning all require an expenditure of energy. They are a productive form of exercise. Second, you are much more likely to eat vegetables and fruit if they come from your own garden, orchard, or vineyard.

A garden can be a steady and reliable source for fresh foods that have much more to offer in the way of taste and nutrition. A vine-ripened tomato, for example, provides much more palate satisfaction than a canned or unripened tomato in a grocery store! Herb gardens can be a good source of fresh herbs, and a flower garden can be a source of non-food rewards!

Gardens feed both the body and soul.

Walk a dog.

❧

*But thinks, admitted to that
equal sky, his faithful dog
shall bear him company.*
—Alexander Pope

On cold winter mornings or hot summer afternoons, the inclination is generally to stay indoors and be comfortable. But there's one member of the household who doesn't have the luxury of choice—the family dog. Use your pet's need to go outside as your excuse to limber up. And if you don't own a dog to walk, consider asking to borrow one from a neighbor.

A dog can make walking, jogging, or running more fun, and in many cases, a dog can provide a measure of safety as you exercise. The companionship of man's best friend can add a whole new dimension to your weight-loss plan.

❧

A dog on a leash can give a new lease on life.

Lose Weight,

I Would . . .

Accept the fact that God loves me from the inside out.

*How great is the love the Father
has lavished on us, that we
should be called children of God.*
—1 John 3:1

God made no perfect body type. He made different heights and structures, noses and foreheads, and He called each one "good." While God desires that you are healthy and fit so that you can better fulfill your potential and purpose in life, He has no requirements for physical perfection, physical health, or physical beauty. He accepts each of us as we are.

Losing weight can allow for easier breathing, increased agility, and an overall better sense of physical appearance, but It will not change your body type, basic facial features, or bone structure. Accept yourself the way God made you, and rest in the fact that God's love is deep and unfaltering.

The most important makeover you can seek is to be transformed into God's spiritual likeness.

If I Really
Wanted to

Lose Weight,

I Would . . .

Start today!

*There is in this world
no such force as a man
determined to rise.*
—W. E. B. Du Bois

January 1 is a date when many people seem to believe all things truly are possible—even the keeping of resolutions that were made the year before and were broken by the first day of February. The best time for changing your life, however, is not the first day of a new year, but today—the first day of the rest of your life.

The dream of losing weight will never be realized unless you make a start. Develop a plan. Set goals. And then work the plan you've made. Patience and hard work are required to reach any worthy goal, but YOU CAN DO IT!

If not now, when?